MSCN EXAM PREPARATION

150 Test Review Questions

**Practice the same number of test questions
as in the actual**

Multiple Sclerosis Nursing International Certification Examination

Adama B. Yansaneh, BSN, RN, MSCN, CCM, CRNI, CCRN, CHC

This book is intended for educational and information purposes only. The book is mostly based on the Author's personal experience in preparing for the Multiple Sclerosis Nursing International Certification Examination. All efforts have been made to verify and clarify the information contained in this book. The Author takes no responsibilities for any omission, errors, or contrary information. The Author makes no expressed or implied warranty or guarantee. The reader assumes all risks in using or taking any advice from this publication.

Dedication

This book is dedicated to people with Multiple Sclerosis and to all the nurses involved in their care, in various capacities, all around the world.

MSCN EXAM PREPARATION

Table of Content

Introduction

The Multiple Sclerosis Nursing International Certification Examination has a maximum of 150 multiple choice type questions and the total testing time is 2.5 hours. The 150 practice questions compiled in this book are formulated in an effort to possibly, indirectly simulate the number and format of questions present in the actual exam. This book is meant to act as a supplemental tool to boost your learning and increase your chances of scoring very high in your certification exam.

Some nursing experts have stated that taking practice tests before actual examinations can prove to be a good test preparation technique. I am a firm believer in that premise and I personally prefer to answer as many practice questions as I can before taking any exam. I usually formulate my own practice questions, and where possible, I use practice questions compiled by expert nurses and other health care professionals.

I have used the Multiple Sclerosis International Certification Examination Handbook for Candidates as a guide to help me prepare the 150 practice questions in this book. These questions are based almost entirely on content areas of the blueprint of the "MSCN Exam," as presented in the Multiple Sclerosis Nursing International Certification Examination Handbook for Candidates.

I wanted to put these 150 practice questions together, because I could not find books or other practice test materials that have a full 150 questions to simulate the number and type of questions present in the actual MSCN exam. I have used information from Multiple Sclerosis books written by other MS health experts to help me compile the practice questions presented in this book.

As a companion to this book, I have also put together a single personal reference book full of exam taking tips, recorded from advice and information I have learnt over the years, on nursing certification test taking techniques.

The title of that book is : Multiple Sclerosis Nursing International Certification Exam: A Step by Step Guide on how to prepare for and Pass the MSCN Exam

I have personally used the skills and techniques outlined in that book, to help me prepare for and pass my various certification exams, each at just one attempt. There are no guarantees in life but, I am hoping that the strategies outlined in that book and the 150 practice questions presented in this one, will be very helpful to other MSCN Exam Candidates, as they were to me, when I took and PASSED my Multiple Sclerosis Nursing International Certification examination, at the very First Attempt.

It is my humble hope that you will find tremendous benefit from using this book as an added study tool for your MSCN exam!

Thank You and Good luck!

Adama B Yansaneh, BSN, RN, MSCN, CCM, CRNI, CCRN, CHC

Contact information: adayans@gmail.com or info@elitecarecorp.com

150 Multiple Sclerosis Nursing Certification Exam Practice Questions

1: What are some common symptoms of Multiple Sclerosis?

A: Generalized weakness, tremors, incoordination, vertigo
B: Focal muscle weakness, fatigue, paresthesias, visual changes
C: Paresthesia, dysarthria, dysphagia, ataxia
D: Vertigo, cognitive dysfunction, tremors, incoordination

#2: What are less common symptoms of Multiple Sclerosis ?

A: Paresthesia, fatigue, bladder dysfunction, depression
B: Neuropathic pain, gait problems, spasticity, depression
C: Ataxia, vertigo, dysphasia, cognitive dysfunction
D: Lhermitte's sign, visual changes, neuropathic pain, fatigue

3: The highest incidence of Multiple Sclerosis is found in people who are:

A: 10 to 59 years of age
B: 20 to 40 years of age
C: 30 to 60 years of age
D: 15 to 45 years of age

#4: The nurse is discussing symptom exacerbation of MS with a 25 year old patient who is planning on getting pregnant. Which statement made by this patient portray's her understanding of the nurse's teaching?

A: Pregnancy can worsen symptom exacerbation in MS Patients.

B: Pregnancy has been known to cause symptom exacerbation and miscarriages in the first trimester .

C: During pregnancy there is about 70% less risk of symptom exacerbation, but the risk will increase again by the same percentage about 3 to 6 months after the baby is born

D: There is no risk of symptom exacerbation during pregnancy.

#5: A patient with advanced MS is having symptoms of ataxic dysarthria and expressive aphasia, the nurse knows that the area of the brain that controls verbal expression is the:

A: Limbic area

B: Pontine area

C: Wernicke area

D: Broca area

#6: A newly diagnosed MS patient had an acute exacerbation during which she incurred a left sided weakness and severe visual changes. You are planning patient teaching with this patient. In talking about the etiology of Multiple Sclerosis you will tell her that MS is classified as a :

A: Demyelinating disorder of the umbilical cord and the spinal cord

B: Motor disorder of the brain and spinal cord

C: Fine motor disorder of the brain and spinal cord

D: Demyelinating disorder of the brain and spinal cord.

#7: **The postulated etiology of Multiple Sclerosis is:**

A: Chemical exposure
B: Chemical imbalance
C: Autoimmune disorder
D: Heredity disorder

#8: **What are the two main types of Multiple Sclerosis?**

A: Relapsing-remitting and Primary-progressive
B: Secondary progressive and Primary resolving
C: Relapsing-remitting and Progressive-remitting
D: Relapsing-resolving and Progressive -resolving

#9: **A 20 year old newly diagnosed Multiple Sclerosis patient says to the nurse: "I hope this diagnoses is wrong. From now on I will exercise, I will eat right, I will change my life style, I pray Lord don't let me have this disease" This behavior is consistent with which stage of Kubler-Ross Model of Grief?**

A: Acceptance
B: Anger
C: Bargaining
D: Denial

#10: **You are performing a neurological assessment on your patient, you know that the Glasgow Coma Scale measures:**

A: Orientation, eye opening and verbal response
B: Orientation, eye opening and motor response
C: Eye opening, verbal response and motor response
D: Orientation, verbal response and activity level

#11: **You measure a total score of 15 on your patient's Glasgow Coma Scale, this score indicates that the patient:**

A: Is in a coma and has no discernible brain function
B: Is physically and neurologically compromised
C: Is likely to be neurologically intact, with minor or no noticeable neurologic deficits
D: Has a very poor chance of survival because of severe brain injury

#12: **Your priority in caring for a patient with advanced stage Multiple Sclerosis is:**

A: Preventions of contractures
B: Prevention of pressure ulcers
C: Prevention of constipation
D: Prevention of aspiration during feedings

#13: **Multiple Sclerosis is diagnosed with which of the following test (s) ?**

A: Cerebrospinal fluids
B: Magnetic Resonance Imaging
C: Evoked Potentials
D: All of the above

#14: **Which of the following would you expect to see in cerebrospinal fluid that has been identified as positive for MS?**

A: Elevated protein and glucose levels.
B: Elevated neutrophil and lymphocyte count.
C: Elevated IgG index or presence of oligoclonal IgG bands in the CSF, but not in serum.
D: Elevated anaerobic or aerobic bacteria in both CSF and serum.

#15: **Lumbar Puncture is contraindicated in which of the following circumstance (s)?**

A: Uncorrected coagulopathy
B: Presence of infected skin at the anatomical area for lumbar puncture
C: Signs of intracranial hemorrhage
D: All of the above

#16: **In which areas of the brain is cerebrospinal fluid formed?**

A: Choroid plexus
B: Arachnoid villi
C: Brain stem
D: Cerebrum

#17: **Your patient is having lumbar puncture done for CSF examination, as the nurse you know that:**

A: Normal Cerebrospinal fluid is clear and colorless. Intrathecal IgG production or presence of oligoclonal igG bands in cerebrospinal fluid but not in serum is an abnormal finding.
B: Some patients may develop headaches, back pain or bleeding post-lumbar puncture.
C: Drinking fluids, lying down, taking over the counter medications like tylenol and NSAIDS for pain management, decrease swelling or fever can be included in your patient teaching.
D: Examining the cerebrospinal fluid is useful when the results of the other tests are not very certain or conclusive.
E: All of the above

#18: In the use of Evoked Potentials for current Multiple Sclerosis diagnosis, which one of the following has been found to be the most useful ?

A: Brainstem Auditory Evoked Potentials (BAEP)
B: Visual Evoked Potentials (VEP)
C: Sensory Evoked Potentials (SEP)
D: None of the above

#19: Which of the following statements about Multiple Sclerosis (MS) is NOT correct?

A: MS is an autoimmune, immune-mediated, inflammatory disease
B: MS is a demyelinating disorder of the Central Nervous System
C: MS is the most common neurological disorder that affects young adults.
D: MS is more prevalent in people of African American descent

#20: Which of the following medications is used to treat walking problems in Multiple Sclerosis?

A: Tizanidine: Zanaflex
B: Vardenafil: Levitra
C: Baclofen: Lioresal
D: Dalfampridine: Ampyra

#21: Fatigue in Multiple Sclerosis is treated with which of the following agents?

A: Modafanil, Armodafinil and Methyphenidate
B: Methylprednisolone, Dexamethasone and H.P. Acthar gel
C: Oxybutinin, Tolterodine, and Fesoterodine
D: Sertraline, Citalopram, Fluoxetine

6

#22: **Natalizumab (Tysabri) is used to treat:**

A: Progressive forms of Multiple Sclerosis
B: Relapsing forms of Multiple Sclerosis
C: Relapsing Progressive forms of Multiple Sclerosis
D: Progressive Remitting forms of Multiple Sclerosis

#23: **Alemtuzumab (Lemtrada) is reserved for use in:**

A: Treatment of relapsing forms of MS that have not had adequate or desired response to two or more MS disease-modifying agents.
B: Relapsing-Remitting MS patients who prefer intravenous medications
C: Patients who want to alternate between Intravenous and subcutaneous MS medications
D: Patients who have progressive forms of Multiple sclerosis

#24: **Which of the following statements is (are) true about Alemtuzumab (Lemtrada) intravenous infusions?**

A: Alemtuzumab is given for five consecutive days initially, followed by three consecutive days one year later. The patients are given corticosteroids and other medications before and after infusions, for management of serious infusion reactions.
B: Patients should have urine and blood work done, before and during treatments, and then every month thereafter, for four or more years after treatment with Alemtuzumab infusions.
C: Patients should be checked for tuberculosis, hepatitis, herpes infections or for history of vaccinations with live vaccines, before starting treatment with Alemtuzumab.
D: Due to the high risk of infusion reactions, autoimmunity and some cancers, Alemtuzumab is given at infusion centers, under a very restricted risk evaluation and mitigation program.
E: All of the above

25: **A Patient with Multiple Sclerosis is to start Natalizumab (Tysabri) infusion. The nurse knows to monitor for which very serious risk factor associated with this medication ?**

A: Chronic Lymphocytic Leukemia
B: Acute anemia
C: Progressive Multifocal Leukoencephalopathy
D: Myocardial Infarction

#26: **A newly diagnosed multiple sclerosis patient who also has diabetes suffered a recent myocardial infarction. During her stay at the hospital, she had episodes of bradycardia and heart block and was further diagnosed with heart failure. Her rubella antibody test is negative. The patient got discharged from the hospital three months ago. The neurologist is planning on getting her started on a disease-modifying agent for her MS. Based on the medical history of this patient, which of the following medications will be contraindicated?**

A: Glatiramer acetate (Copaxone)
B: Fingolimod hydrochloride (Gilenya)
C: Betaseron (Interferon Beta-1b)
D: Plegridy (Peginterferon Beta-1a)

#27: **A newly married 25 year old female with relapsing form of MS tells you she is planning on having children as soon as possible. She asks you questions about the safety of some disease-modifying agents during pregnancy. Per FDA pregnancy category of medications, which of the following agents is comparably less risky for use in pregnancy?**

A: Natalizumab (Tysabri)
B: Dimythyl fumarate (Tecfidera)
C: Glatiramer acetate (Copaxone)
D: Alemtuzumab (Lemtrada)

#28: **All of the following classes of medication are used to manage pain in MS except:**

A: PDE-5 inhibitors
B: Muscle relaxants
C: Tricyclic antidepressants
D: Anticonvulsants

#29: **Which of the following medications are used for treatment in the chronic phase of Trigeminal neuralgia?**

A: Oxycodone and Percocet
B: Tylenol, Aspirin and Advil
C: Gabapentin and carbamazepine,
D: Baclofen and morphine sulfate

#30: **All the following are true about symptom management in MS except:**

A: Baclofen can be used in trigeminal neuralgia, spasticity or painful tonic spasms
B: Phenytoin is good for managing dysesthetic or abnormal, unpleasant sensations.
C: Misoprostol can be prescribed for MS symptom management in pregnant patients.
D: Acute Trigeminal Neuralgia can be treated with IV or oral steroids
E: Lhermittes's sign can be treated with anti-seizure and tricyclic antidepressants medications.

#31: **Which one of the following immunosuppressant agents is approved for use in the treatment of worsening forms of Multiple Sclerosis?**

A: Azathioprine
B: Mitoxantrone
C: Cyclophosphamide
D: None of the above

#32: **Abrupt withdrawal of intrathecal Baclofen can result in which of the following ?**

A: Altered mental status
B: High fever
C: Exaggerated rebound spasticity
D: Muscle rigidity
E: All of the above

#33: **The nurse has just completed injection training with a patient on Glatiramer actetate The patient verbalized understanding of the training information and performed accurate return demonstration of injection techniques. Within 10 minutes after getting the initial injection, the patient becomes anxious and starts complaining of chest pain, dyspnea and a general feeling of warmth. The nurse knows that:**

A: The patient is having a cardiac event and needs immediate medical attention.

B: The patient should chew four aspirin tablets and then call 911.

C: These symptoms are rare, they lasts for about 15 minutes and do not usually need specific medical treatment.

D: The patient should call the emergency phone number if the symptoms persist or become worse.

E: Both C and D

#34: **Which of the following are common side effects of Glatriramer Acetate?**

A: Redness, pain, itching, or swelling at the injection site

B: Fever, pain, shivering, flu like symptoms

C: Abdominal pain, diarrhea, nausea, vomiting

D: Increased liver enzymes, headaches, nausea

#35: **A 35 year old female patient with a history of multiple relapses since she was first diagnosed two years ago, had recent treatment with both oral and intravenous steroids at the nearby local hospital.** The patient is now wondering why the steroid treatments are not getting her relapsing form of MS healed well enough to avoid any further relapse.
The nurse knows that:

A: Corticosteroids and glucocorticoids (Steroids) help shorten the duration of relapses but they do not change the course of the disease.

B: MethlyPrednisolone (medrol) is an oral glucocorticoid.

C: Methylprednisolone sodium succinate is an intravenous adrenal glucocorticoid.

D: H.P. Acthar can be given IM or SUBQ.

E: All of the above

#36: **Which of the following are oral disease-modifying agents?**

A: Betaseron, Extavia Rebif

B: Tecfidera, Aubagio, Gilenya

C: Lemtrada, Novantrone, Tysabri

D: Copaxone, Avonex, Plegridy

#37: **Side effects associated with Interferon beta 1-a and 1-b (intramuscular and subcutaneous) agents include all of the following except:**

A: Flu-like symptoms

B: Injection site skin reactions

C: Elevated liver enzymes

D: Nausea, vomiting, diarrhea, bladder dysfunction and loss of appetite

#38: **Which of the following agents are classified as Interferon beta-1a ?**

A: Copaxone and Glatopa
B: Plegridy, Avonex and Rebif
C: Betaseron and Extavia
D: None of the above

#39: **Which of the following agents are classified as antidepressants?**

A: Fluoxetine, Paroxetine, Sertraline, Escitalopram
B: Oxybutinin, Tolterodine, Denifenacin, Hycoscyamine
C: Sildenafil, Tadalafil, Vardenafil
D: Diazepam, Clonazepam, Imipramine

#40: **A 44 year old female with relapsing remitting form of MS has an increase in anti -JCV antibodies and her liver enzymes are elevated. Her oral disease modifying agent, Tecfidera, is being changed to Glatiramer subcutaneous injections. The patient is concerned that she may not be able to learn the injection techniques for the new medication.The best educational strategies to help this patient learn the injection techniques would be:**

A: Have a nurse arrange a visit with the patient to teach her how to administer the injections.
B: Have the patient go to the manufacturer's website and learn how to do the injections on her own, when she has enough free time to focus.
C: Use video materials and written instructions.
D: Have the nurse call the patient and teach her the injection techniques over the phone.
E: A and C

#41: **When teaching side effect management for injectable agents, the nurse will do patient and family education on all of the following except:**

A: Appropriate injection sites and importance of site rotation

B: Dose titration and timing of injections, as indicated

C: NSAID drugs and lab work, as indicated

D: Tell the patient to take periodic medication holidays when side effects occur.

#42: **Barriers to medication adherence can be caused by which of the following ?**

A: Patient's age

B: Knowledge deficit

C: Financial problems

D: Alternate cultural beliefs

E: B, C, D

#43: **Your patient was placed on Elavil, for depression, one week ago. The patient is severely depressed and the family is becoming frustrated. The husband asks you why the patient has remained depressed even though she has been on an anti depressant for a whole week. As the nurse you know that:**

A: The patient needs a different anti depressant

B: Tricyclic antidepressants may take a few weeks to show symptomatic improvement in patients.

C: The dose of the Elavil may need to be increased for this patient.

D: The patient has already built a tolerance to Elavil.

#44: **Your MS patient who is suffering from bladder dysfunction is requesting information about treatment for some bladder disorder symptoms. As the nurse you know that:**

A: Urinary urgency and frequency can be treated with Oxybutinin, Fesoterodine, Tolterodine and Denifenacin

B: Urinary urgency and frequency can be treated with Tamsulosin and Tofranil

C: Urinary hesitancy/retention can be treated with Tamsulosin and Terazosin

D: A and C

E: A and B

#45: **A 25 year old newly married MS patient, who is planning on having children, is concerned about the well being of her potential unborn fetus, now that she has been diagnosed with MS and has to take disease-modifying agents. As the MS nurse you know that all of the following are true except:**

A: Pregnancy and the immediate postpartum are the periods when MS relapse rates are very prevalent and dangerous for both mother and fetus.

B: Currently, there is no credible research evidence to support the notion that MS disease itself can directly harm an unborn child.

C: Interferon- beta medications like Avonex, Betaseron and Rebif are FDA Pregnancy Category C

D: Glatiramer acetate is a Pregnancy Category B drug, a lower risk than interferons, but risk/benefit ratio should be considered when using any of these medications during pregnancy.

#46: **Your patient is taking Sildenafil citrate to manage his sexual dysfunction, which one of the following medication class is (are) contraindicated in this case?**

A: Tricyclic anti depressants and benzodiazepines
B: Interferon 1-a and 1-b
C: Organic nitrates and Protease inhibitors
D: Benzodiazepines and NSAIDS

#47: **You are reviewing medications with a patient with relapsing form of MS. She was on Copaxone 20 mg, but her new health insurance is considering changing the Copaxone to Glatopa 20 mg to save on cost. The patient tells you she is not very familiar with this new medication. She thinks the "new medication might be a pill form" but she is not sure. As the MS nurse you know that:**

A: Glatopa 20 mg is a subcutaneous injection used to treat Relapsing forms of Multiple Sclerosis.
B: Glatopa 20mg is the generic form of Copaxone / Glatiramer acetate 20mg
C: Most common side effects of Glatiramer acetate include, pain, swelling, itching and burning sensations at injection sites.
D: a, b and c

#48: **Which one of the following statements is not correct ?**

A: Liver function test, CBC with differential and other blood chemistry tests are recommended during therapy with Interferon beta agents.

B: Betaseron and Extavia are interferon 1-b immunosuppressant agents.

C: Plegridy (Peginterferon beta 1-a) can cause serious side effects that include liver problems, worsening depressions and suicidal thoughts.

D: Unlike Tysabri (Natalizumab) patients taking Tecfidera (Dimethyl Fumarate) have no risk of getting PML (Progressive Multifocal leukoencephalopathy)

#49: **You are performing teaching with a patient whose medication has been changed from Betaseron to Glatiramer acetate. As the nurse, you know that a major difference between the Interferons and Glatiramer acetate is:**

A: Glatiramer acetate causes elevated liver enzymes and decreased white blood cells

B: Betaseron is effective in Primary progressive MS

C: Interferons are associated with flu-like symptoms, Glatiramer acetate is not associated with flu-like symptoms.

D: Patients on Glatiramer acetate need monitoring for laboratory abnormalities

#50: **Your patient is having problems with bowel and bladder incontinence, she begins to cry and says "This must be why my husband does not want to be intimate with me anymore." Which of the following should be the initial action of the nurse?**

A: Make arrangements to speak with the husband
B: Refer the couple to a marriage counsellor
C: Explore the patient's feelings
D: Tell the patient it will be better for her to focus on getting treatment for her symptoms first, then worry about intimacy with her husband later.

#51: **Which of the following statements about Multiple Sclerosis is incorrect?**

A: MS is a progressive, neurodegenerative inflammatory disease of the Central Nervous System.
B: MS is a demyelinating disease of the Central Nervous System that mainly affects the white matter.
C: MS is a demyelinating disease of the Peripheral Nervous System that mainly affects the grey matter.
D: MS is a chronic autoimmune, inflammatory, demyelinating disease that has no absolute, confirmed, definitive cause at this time.

#52: **The possible causes of MS are postulated to be which of the following statements ?**

A: Demyelination of myelin sheaths, destruction of axons, multiple scarring in the Central Nervous System
B: Chronic autoimmune response to environmental triggers in genetically predisposed patients
C: Abnormal autoimmune response to a combination of triggers, from viruses or other components found in the environment, geographic locations, race or gender in genetically predisposed patients.
D: Immune system activation of white blood cells
E: All of the above

#53: **According to the Multiple Sclerosis foundation, statistically**

A: More than 400,000 people in the United States and approximately 2.5 million people around the world have MS.
B: About 200, 000 people in the United States and 5.2 million people around the world have MS.
C: About 2.5 million people in the United States and 10 million people around the world have MS.
D: 4 million people in the United States and 16 million people around the world have MS.

#54: **Multiple Sclerosis is more prevalent in:**

A: Women than in men
B: In Caucasians than in none Caucasians
C: In temperate, colder areas than in warmer climate areas
D: All of the above

#55: **You are performing an initial assessment on your MS patient, as you firmly stroke the sole of her foot, you notice dorsiflexion of her big toe, while her other toes fan outwards. You interpret this finding as a:**

A: Negative Babinski response
B: Positive Babinski response
C: Positive Romberg test
D: Negative Romberg test

#56: **A positive Babinski reflex indicates:**

A: A normal neurologic finding
B: Upper motor neuron lesions of the corticospinal tract
C: Lower and middle motor lesions of the pyramidal tract
D: Both upper and lower lesions of the pyramidal tract

#57: **Charcot's neurologic triad in MS is defined as:**

A: Lhermittes sign, ataxia and dystonia.
B: Nystagmus, dysarthria and intension tremors.
C: Bladder dysfunction, sexual dysfunction and cognitive dysfunction
D: Constipation, bloating and abdominal pain

#58: **Which of the following is (are) true about Uhthoff's Phenomenon?**

A: Uhthoff phenomenon refers to a rise in core body temperature from exercise, hot weather, stress or other heat related issues, that lead to visual and other worsening MS symptoms.

B: Is also referred to as pseudoexacerbation, not a true MS relapse.

C: It can be controlled by using cooling equipment and other cooling strategies, during the summer heat especially.

D: All of the above

#59: **When teaching a patient how to reduce fatigue in MS, during the summer months especially, the nurse should tell the patient to:**

A: Stay in air conditioned rooms or use other cooling agents

B: Take warm showers in the afternoons

C: Ask the doctor to increase the dose of her muscle relaxers

D: Avoid day time naps

#60: **Oligodendrocytes are the actual cells:**

A: That produce Schwann cells and dendrites

B: That produce the axon and the cell body of neurons

C: That create the myelin sheaths, which provide support and insulation for axons

D: That produce the white blood cells, which destroys myelin sheaths

#61: **Clinically isolated symptoms (CIS) can be:**

A: The first episode of neurologic symptom that lasts for at least 24 hours
B: Caused by inflammation or demyelination in the CNS
C: A monofocal or multifocal episode
D: The patient has no fever or infection
E: All of the Above

#62: **A patient with MS has been complaining of jabbing, spontaneous, excruciating pain to her face and her jaws when she does simple things such as brushing her teeth or touching her face to put on make- up. As the nurse, you recognize these symptoms as a problem in MS that is associated with:**

A: Cranial Nerve V- Trigeminal Nerve
B: Cranial Neve X- Vagus Nerve
C: Cranial Nerve VIII- Acoustic Nerve
D: Cranial Nerve II - Optic Nerve

#63: **When teaching about the prevention of pain in Trigeminal Neuralgia, which of the following is the most appropriate instruction to give to your patient?**

A: Avoid Brushing your teeth every day
B: Chew on the unaffected side
C: Chew Ice chips at meal times
D: Apply warm compress at bedtime

#64: **Relapsing-remitting form of Multiple Sclerosis is diagnosed in about what percentage of patients?**

A: 25%
B: 50%
C: 85%
D: 20%

#65: **Which of the following information is (are) true about Primary progressive MS (PPMS)**

A: PPMS is diagnosed in approximately 15% of MS patients, it is more difficult to diagnose and treat than RRMS.
B: PPMS is marked by slow, steady, worsening, declining neurologic function, without periods of relapses and remissions like in RRMS.
C: In PPMS increased problems with walking and other disabilities interfere with the everyday activities of people.
D: Unlike RRMS where seventy to seventy five percent of patients are female, in PPMS the ratio of male to female is about equal.
E: All of the above

#66: **A 35 year old female with optic neuritis was admitted to the hospital three weeks ago for management of MS symptom exacerbation. Since she was diagnosed two years ago, she has had two other exacerbations, both of which she recovered from fully. During her admission, she was treated with high-dose Intravenous Methylprednisolone sodium succinate, then she was discharged home, after her symptoms were fully resolved. As the MS nurse, you know that this patient most likely has:**

A: Progressive-relapsing MS
B: Relapsing-remitting MS
C: Secondary-progressing MS
D: Primary-progressive MS

#67: **Which of the following statement (s) about relapse in MS is (are) correct?**

A: A relapse is the occurrence of a new symptom or the reoccurrence of previous MS symptoms.
B: A relapse must lasts for a period of over 24 hours.
C: A relapse must not be related to an infection or an environmental factor.
D: Relapses can be managed with high-dose steroids for defined, limited periods of time.
E: All of the above.

#68: **When caring for a patient with Relapsing-remitting MS, which one of the following intervention (s) will the nurse include?**

A: Make sure the patient has access to disease-modifying agents.
B: Ensure that the patient is using appropriate techniques for medication administration.
C: Emphasize the importance of adherence to medication / treatment regimen.
D: Instruct the patient to avoid excessive temperatures, infections and fevers, to help minimize MS symptom exacerbation.
E: All of the above

#69: **Exacerbation in Multiple Sclerosis includes which of the following list of symptoms?**

A: Urinary incontinence, constipation or bowel dysfunction
B: Diplopia, emotional lability or ataxia
C: Dementia, ataxia, or paresthesia
D: Delirium, trigeminal neuralgia or sexual dysfunction

#70: **Nursing education for the prevention and control of Pseudoexacerbations include:**

A: Promotion of hand hygiene, avoidance of infection, fevers or increase in core body temperature.
B: Use of cooling devices, hydration with cool drinks and maintaining cool, ambient temperature.
C: Exercising in cool areas; avoidance of over heating, wearing light clothing, drinking cool drinks during exercise.
D: All of the above

#71: **A 20 year old college student who has been diagnosed with relapsing form of MS is to start treatment with an injectable disease- modifying agent. The patient wants to know why she should take these injections so early in her disease course, when she is not even having severe symptoms yet. Your patient teaching will be based on all of the following except:**

A: Disease-modifying agents help reduce relapse severity.
B: Relapse rates may be fewer when disease-modifying agents are started early.
C: Disease-modifying agents help delay progression of disability.
D: MS symptoms are eliminated when disease-modifying agents are started early.

#72: **You have a referral to visit a patient who has not been taking her medications as prescribed and scheduled. You would implement all of the following nursing actions except:**

A: Include family and support persons during medication teaching to improve adherence.
B: Include video and written materials in your patient teaching.
C: Give the patient information about 24 hour nursing telephone support.
D: Make decisions for the patient about her treatment and medication regimen.

#73: **Which of the following statements is (are) true about MRI results in the diagnosis of Multiple Sclerosis ?**

A: T1 dark spots / black holes, hypointense lesions on MRI, may reflect edema resulting from severe demyelination, damaged myelin coating, destroyed nerve fibers and axons. Chronic T1 "black holes" indicate more severe damaged brain tissue, that may put patients at higher risk for physical disability.
B: T1-weighted MRI images may give information about disease activity by identifying areas of edema or active inflammation. The swelling may be temporary, it may come and go, or it may not show up in follow-up MRIs. The edema may be the result of damaged brain tissue.
C: T2 -weighted images are hyperintense lesions that show up as bright, white spots on MRI. They are the result of demyelination, hypertrophic glial cells, damaged matrix or edema.
D: T2 lesion load refers to the entire amount of lesions, both old and new. The total number or volume of lesions on MRI images may reflect the MS disease burden. MS patients with larger numbers of T2 lesions are at increase risk for disability.
E: All of the above

#74: **Which of the following statements is (are) associated with the Revised McDonald diagnostic criteria for MS ?**

A: **Dissemination in Time (DIT) and Space (DIS)** are terms or descriptions used, during the MRI diagnostic process of MS, to show the presence of demyelinating lesions or damage, occurring within a period of time, in specific locations in the CNS.

B: Proof of **Dissemination in Space (DIS)** is when there is evidence of T2 lesions located at a minimum of two of these four areas of the CNS, namely: the spinal cord, the periventricular, the infratentorial and the juxtacortical spaces.

C: **Dissemination In Time (DIT)** is when asymptomatic gadolinuem -enhancing lesions or non enhancing lesions are present at any time, or new T2 lesions are noticed in a follow up MRI, as compared to a previous MRI, that was done within a month of the first known clinical attack.

D: In the presence of a clinical attack, an MRI result that has T2 weighted lesions present in the periventricular white matter, brain stem and spinal cord can be considered positive.

E: All of the above

#75: **Criteria for diagnosing Multiple Sclerosis include which of the following?**

A: Two or more attacks, with at least one clinical confirmed lesion, occurring in at least two separate MS known areas of the Central Nervous System (CNS).

B: A new T2 lesion occurring at any time, in a follow up MRI, as compared to a baseline, reference MRI scan, that was done within 30 days of the onset of the first known clinical signs.

C: The possibility of other causes are ruled out.

D: One clinical attack, a positive CSF and two or more MRI lesions in areas of the CNS that are known for MS injury occurrence.

E: All of the above

#76: Which one of the following statements is not true about MRI and the Blood Brain Barrier?

A: During MRIs, Gadolinium contrast is used to show areas of acute inflammation or damage.

B: Gadolinium is able to cross an intact blood-brain barrier.

C: A breakdown in the blood brain barrier can predispose the brain and spinal cord tissues to attack and injury from inflammatory cells.

D: When breakdown occurs in the blood- brain barrier, inflammatory immune cells are able to invade the brain parenchyma.

#77: All of the following statements about MS are true except:

A: In MS, a breakdown of the usually intact blood-brain barrier occurs, causing migration of lymphocytes, macrophages and other immune system cells in to the Central Nervous System.

B: Currently, the diagnoses of MS is a clinical one; there is no single, definitive diagnostic laboratory test for the disease.

C: In MS, persistent inflammation, demyelination and scarring can lead to permanent axonal destruction and loss.

D: Axonal damage and loss can occur in the early stages of MS, even before clinical signs and symptoms are noticed or reported.

E: Disease-modifying, immunemodulating and immunosuppressive agents can reverse the damage and destruction done to axonal nerve fibers and brain tissues in MS.

#78: **Which of the following statements is (are) true about Lhermitte's sign?**

A: Lhermitte's sign is a sudden electrical sensation, pain or paresthesia that runs down the back on to the legs or arms of patients.
B: Lhermitte's sign can occur when the neck is flexed or bent, resulting in a sudden sensation that can travel from the neck to the spine.
C: Lhermitte's sign can be managed with medications, posture monitoring and relaxation techniques..
D: Lhermitte's sign can suggest demyelination, lesions in the caudal medulla or dorsal columns of the cervical cord.
E: All of the above

#79: **Which of the following will less likely increase the intensity of MS symptoms during hot Summer months?**

A: Use of ceiling fans or air conditioning
B: Hot or humid environment
C: Infections and fevers
D: None compliance with prescribed disease modifying agents

#80 : **Which of the following actions would be the best intervention to help manage MS symptoms in warm environments?**

A: Walking outside for exercise
B: Taking a warm shower
C: Use of air conditioners or other cooling methods.
D: Getting adequate sleep

#81: **When assessing a patient with multiple sclerosis, a primary finding is:**

A: Visual changes like nystagmus or diplopia,
B: Pressure ulcer on the sacrum
C: Severe abdominal pain
D: Unplanned Weight loss of 15 pounds in the last one month

#82: **Which of the following is (are) true about the use of glucocorticoids and corticosteroids (steroids) in MS?**

A: Some side effects of steroid medications are thirst, heartburn, dyspnea and palpitations
B: Relapses are managed with intravenous or oral steroid agents
C: Steroid medications are used for a limited period of time; chronic steroid use is not recommended.
D: Corticosteroids and glucocorticoids can shorten periods of MS symptom exacerbation.
E: All of the above

#83: **Problems with tremors, asthenia and ataxia are related to the :**

A: Brain stem
B: Optic nerve
C: Peripheral nerves
D: Sensory pathways

#84: **Which of the following definitions of conditions in MS is (are) correct?**

A: Nystagmus: is an abnormal involuntary, uncontrolled, repetitive eye movement, that can cause problems with depth perception, gait disturbance, balance and coordination in MS.

B: Abnormal, positive Babinski reflex is: when firm stroking of the lateral side of the sole of the foot, results in upward extension of the big toe, and fanning out of the other toes.

C: Optic Neuritis: a key finding in MS, is the Inflammation of the nerve fibers in the optic nerve, the main areas that transmit visual information to our brains.

D: Molecular mimicry: Is when foreign antigens and the host/self-peptides share similar molecular structures. It is the process where the immune system, which usually reacts to foreign antigens, now reacts against and destroys myelin, a component of the self.

E: All of the above

#85: A **65 year old multiple sclerosis patient shares her home with her 35 year old unemployed son. During your nursing assessment, you notice some bruising on her face and arms. The Patient will not tell you what happened to her when the son is in the room.**
Your initial nursing action would be to:

A: Talk to the Patient and her son about the bruises.

B: Notify the authorities about the bruises and the abuse.

C: Talk to the Patient about the bruises when the son is not present.

D: Do nothing because the bruises are not caused by her MS.

#86: **Demyelination, scarring and destruction of nerve fibers that occur in MS can lead to which of the following symptoms?**

A: Dysarthria, dysphagia, ataxia, vertigo, and paresthesia
B: Fatigue, focal weakness, depression and tremors
C: Constipation, incoordination, sexual dysfunction, bowel and bladder dysfunction
D: Neuritic pain, Lhermitte's sign, spasticity, and cognitive difficulties
E: All of the above

#87: **Which of the following statements about MS patients is not true?**

A: Having supportive and satisfying relationships is critical for MS patients.
B: There is variability in the course of the disease, from one individual to another.
C: In general, MS occurs in more women than men.
D: The average age of onset in MS is 30 to 60 years

#88: **You are providing care for four MS patients this week, which one of these four patients would you say has the worst prognosis?**

A: 42 year old year old female, who was diagnosed at age 22, had mono regional attacks, has been pregnant twice, had one relapse last year, from which she recovered very well.

B: 40 year old female, diagnosed at age 20, recovered well from her first relapse and has had very long intervals between her relapses.

C: 50 year old male, who was diagnosed at age 40, his MRI had very high lesion load. He has high relapse rate and and is still recovering from left sided weakness and other symptoms he incurred in the last relapse, 3 years ago.

D: 50 year old female, was diagnosed at age 21, she recovered from her first relapse but started developing some mild problems with walking just this year.

#89: **Respecting and supporting the rights, culture, values and beliefs of your MS patient is called?**

A: Moral duty
B: legal duty
C: Standard of care
D: Advocacy

#90: **Your patient is complaining of having bladder related problems. He is not able to empty his bladder properly and he has issues with storing urine. You suspect the patient has bladder dysfunction. As the nurse you know that the common cause (s) of bladder dysfunction is (are) :**

A: Detrusor areflexia or problems with relaxation and opening of the sphincter
B: Lack of coordination of the detrusor and sphincter activity also known as Detrusor sphincter dyssynergia (DSD)
C: Increased contractility of the detrusor muscle
D: All of the above

#91: **Nursing assessment of a patient with bladder dysfunction includes which of the following?**

A: Evaluating and confirming patient's chief complaint
B: Taking a history of patient's voiding patterns, including periods of urinary incontinence, urgency, frequency and other urinary problems
C: Evaluating post void residual volume with bladder scan or straight catheter
D: Checking patient's current medications.
E: All of the above

#92: **Which of the following statement (s) indicate problems with bladder dysfunction?**

A: The need to urinate every 2 to 3 hours (urinary frequency)
B: Very strong, uncontrolled urge to urinate (urinary urgency)
C: Difficulty starting urine flow (urinary hesitancy)
D: Lack of control of urine (Incontinence)
E: All of the above

#93: **While performing a bowel and bladder function assessment on your patient, she tells you that for the past one year, she has used over-the-counter laxatives every week, to help promote bowel regularity. As the nurse you know that excessive use of laxatives can put patients at risk for:**

    A: Diarrhea
    B: Abdominal bloating
    C: Chronic constipation
    D: Abdominal distention

#94: **In a patient experiencing bowel dysfunction, the nurse would give all of the following instructions except:**

A: Increase your intake of fluids and fiber
B: Use stool softeners and glycerine suppositories
C: Don't worry, diarrhea happens in MS frequently
D: Sit in an upright position on the toilet with your feet on the floor

95: **Which of the following statements about depression is (are) correct?**

A: Newly diagnosed, younger age females are at very high risk for depression
B: Disease activity and reaction to difficult life changes can cause depression
C: Treatment for depression include medications, psychotherapy, counseling and emotional support.
D: Neuroendocrine or psychoneuroimmunologic changes can lead to depression in MS
E: All of the above

#96: All of the following statements are true about depression in MS patients except:

A: Suicide rate is higher in MS than in the general populations
B: Newly diagnosed, young female patients have higher risk for depression than others
C: Some common agents used to treat depressions are Fluoxetine, Paroxetine, Sertraline and Amitriptyline.
D: Depression is not commonly seen in patients with Multiple Sclerosis

#97: Your newly diagnosed MS patient has had increased mood changes in the last few weeks. She is very withdrawn and has started giving her belongings away to strangers. In your assessment of this patient, which of the following behaviors show a possible sign of suicidal ideation?

A: The Patient is frequently asking for medications for anxiety and depression.
B: The Patient is constantly staying in her room and does not want to interact with others.
C: The Patient isolates herself, she cries increasingly and describes herself as a hopeless, worthless, useless person, whom nobody loves or cares about.
D: The Patient is yelling and arguing with her relatives in your presence.

#98: A patient who is exhibiting sadness, has pessimistic thinking, lowered self-esteem and guilt may be suffering from which of the following?

A: Delirium
B: Dementia
C: Depression
D: Paranoia

#99: **All of the following are true about cognitive changes in MS except:**

A: Cognitive changes in MS can be linked to the root cause of the disease itself or to other secondary effects of the condition.

B: Primary effects can be attributed to cerebral demyelination, axonal nerve cell damage ,and variability of multi focal lesions.

C: Possible secondary causes of cognitive changes are anxiety, depression, fatigue and stress.

D: Severe cognitive changes are very common in MS

#100: **When assessing patients for cognitive changes the nurse knows that:**

A: The inability to remember, think or reason logically are all features seen in the clinical setting.

B: Verbal fluency, timing of information processing, problem solving and abstract reasoning can all be affected by cognitive changes

C: Cognitive impairment can affect a patent's family, social and work life

D: A, B and C

#101: **Nursing interventions in cognitive changes include:**

A: Recognizing and acknowledging the patient's cognitive deficits

B: Accurately reporting and documenting evaluation results

C: Establishing a supportive patient and family relationships

D: Promoting appropriate coping strategies and safe environments

E: All of the above

#102: Your **MS** patient's husband tells you that he is surprised his wife can remember things from their early life together, but has become very forgetful of everyday, recent events. You are not surprise, because you know that in MS the least likely cognitive function to be affected is:

A: Information processing
B: Attention and Concentration
C: Long-term memory
D: Recall memory

#103: **Nursing education of patients with cognitive impairment should include all of the following except:**

A: Repeating information and facilitating communication
B: Recognizing deficits and promoting coping strategies
C: Providing teaching in quiet, familiar environments to patient
D: Have music playing in the background during teaching

104: **Which of the following MS patients has a better disease prognosis?**

A: Female ,with disease onset at age 24, with monoregional attacks, has been pregnant once.
B: Male, with disease onset at age 50, has dysarthria, ataxia and tremors.
C: 45 year old male, with polyregional attacks, had poor recovery after his first relapse episode.
D: 45 year old female with brain stem and cerebella symptoms.

#105: **When providing care for a patient with advanced MS, the nurse should be alert for which of the following potential problem (s) ?**

A: Swallowing difficulties
B: Depression
C: Pressure ulcers
D: All of the above

#106: **When providing nursing care and patient education for clients with advanced MS, the nurse knows to include which of the following?**

A: Discussion of the use of corticosteroids
B: Providing palliative care as needed
C: Implementing interventions to prevent pressure ulcers
D: All of the above

#107: **You are caring for a patient who has advanced MS, as the nurse you would do which of the following?**

A: Discuss Advanced Directives
B: Encourage life planning, education and counseling
C: Allow opportunities for families to communicate their fears and concerns
D: a, b, and c

#108: **All of the following statements about sexual dysfunction in MS are true except:**

A: Primary sexual dysfunction can result from MS-related physiologic changes in the Central Nervous System.

B: Secondary sexual dysfunction is caused by MS- related physical changes like depression, pain, fatigue, tremors, nongenital sensory paresthesia.

C: Erectile dysfunction can be managed with Levitra, Cialis and Viagra.

D: Men and women MS patients can have similar pharmacological management for sexual dysfunction.

#109: **In providing care for a Multiple Sclerosis patient with sexual dysfunction problems, the nurse should :**

A: Find out what the patient's values, beliefs and attitudes towards sex are.

B: Allow privacy and a nonjudgemental atmosphere.

C: Validate the patient's concerns and make referrals to appropriate resources, as indicated.

D: Use open-ended questions and offer support as needed.

E: All of the above

#110: **Which of the following statements is (are) true about pediatric MS?**

A: It is less readily diagnosed than in adult populations

B: It can present with fever, listlessness and other systemic symptoms

C: There is very little likelihood of abnormal changes in the cerebrospinal fluid

D: Diagnostic markers may not be the same as in adults

E: all of the above

#111: **A 45 year old female with a history of chronic renal diseases is scheduled to have MRI (magnetic resonance imaging) with gadolinium /IV contrast. The result of which of the following lab tests should be known prior to giving the IV contrast to this patient?**

A: White Blood Cells
B: Prothrombin Time
C: Creatinine
D: Hematocrit

#112: **When providing care for MS patients who use complimentary and alternative therapies, the nurse knows that these non-conventional therapies include all of the following except:**

A: Hypnosis, meditation and spiritual connections
B: Diets, herbal and mineral supplements
C: Massage, acupuncture and chiropractic therapies
D: Acetaminophen, Motrin and Advil

#113: **The Nurse's role in working with a patient who is using complementary/ alternative therapy include:**

A: Enquiring about the kind of herbs and supplements the patient is using.
B: Providing information and teaching about the risk of combining traditional drugs with contraindicated non-conventional treatments.
C: Giving the patient information about appropriate resources, as applicable
D: a, b, & c

#114: **When providing education and care to MS patients, the nurse should:**

A: Have Knowledge about Multiple Sclerosis disease
B: Use Nursing theories and the Nursing Process, as applicable
C: Utilize principles of teaching and learning, as applicable
D: a, b & c

115: **The Nurse as a patient advocate would:**

A: Be a disease expert and spread MS disease awareness
B: Empower patients, protect patient's rights
C: Be a patient consultant and serve as a negotiator for patients and their families
D: Promote and advocate for appropriate self-care strategies
E: All of the above

#116: **Which of the following statements about MS is not true?**

A: In MS, demyelinated lesions are of varying age, disseminated in location, but are most evident in the white matter than the grey matter of the CNS
B: Inflammation, demyelination, scarring in the CNS eventually results in damage to oligodendrocytes and axons.
C: Slow, delayed, conduction failures can all occur in demyelinated nerve fibers.
D: The etiology of MS is without any doubt related to viral, environmental and immune- mediated factors.

#117: **The domains of MS nursing practice include:**

A: Clinical practice, advocacy, education and research
B: Assessment, planning, diagnosis, implementation and evaluation
C: Denial, anger, bargaining, depression and acceptance
D: Physiological, safety, love/belonging, esteem and self-actualization

#118: **The World Health Organization has defined a person's functional abilities as:**

A: Disability
B: Activity Level
C: Chandicaps
D: Mobility

#119: **Clinical course of MS includes which one of the following?**

A: Relapsing-remitting MS (RRMS)
B: Secondary- progressive MS (SPMS)
C: Primary- progressive MS (PPMS)
D: Progressive-relapsing MS (PRMS)
E: All of the above

#120 : **Which of the following statements is not true?**

A: Numbness, paresthesias, Lhermitte's sign are common sensory presentations in MS.
B: Motor abnormalities in MS include spasticity, limb weakness, heaviness and positive Babinski reflex.
C: Visual problems in MS include diplopia, nystagmus and optic neuritis.
D: Major causes of MS symptoms are decreased production of white blood cells, cytokines and other inflammatory cells in the Central Nervous System.

#121: **A nurse is performing an assessment on a client involved in Multiple Sclerosis research, which of the following would the nurse be expected to look for?**

A: How realistic the patient's expectations are about what the study drug will do or not do.
B: How committed the patient is to following the testing requirements, procedures, and number of visits outlined in the protocol and consent form.
C: How well the patient has adhered to treatments or other study appointments in the past?
D: a,b & c

#122: **Which of the following statements about adherence is not correct?**

A: A patient's cultural beliefs can influence medication and treatment adherence.
B: Adequate information and support can improve adherence.
C: Adequate knowledge and patient satisfaction can influence adherence.
D: To promote adherence, nurses and other health care professionals should make treatment decisions for patients.

#123: **Neuropsychological evaluation is appropriate in which of the following?**

A: A family member is worried that a patient probably has some cognitive deficit, the patient denies it and she has shown no notable physical or clinical evidence.

B: A boss at work is concerned that a patient has started dressing slovenly to work and her work quality has deteriorated in the last month.

C: A patient is concerned that she is having cognitive deficits that occasionally affect her day to day function..

D: A newly diagnosed MS patient who is concerned and worried about starting treatment with immunosuppressive agents.

E: All of the above

#124: **During medication injection training, you notice multiple bruises on the arms and neck of your patient. You suspect possible physical abuse. Which of the following indicators would most support your assessment?**

A: The patient hesitates to discuss her home situation

B: The patient willingly volunteers information

C: The patient quickly and abruptly denies abuse when asked directly

D: The patient is showing more extroverted behavior

#125: **A patient needs to make some treatment decision but does not yet have enough information and knowledge to do so. The nurse experiences conflict and feels obligated to assist the patient in making the decisions.**
This kind of behavior is known as:

A: Codependency
B: Paternalism
C: Moral guidance
D: Constructive thinking

#126: **In many none Western families, cultural values and practices most likely include which of the following beliefs ?**

A: Disease is caused by disagreement with others
B: Decisions must be made by patients only
C: Medicinal herbs and non-traditional treatments are very useful
D: Western medicine is not good

#127: **A Patient with MS is having problems with coordination and balance. As the nurse you know that theses symptoms are related to problems in the :**

A: The cerebrum
B: The cerebellum
C: The brain stem
D: The spinal cord

#128: **When providing care for a patient who is complaining of fatigue, the nurse would teach the patient to do all of the following except:**

A: Get at least 8 hours of sleep, have frequent breaks and regular rest periods
B: Increase your caffein intake to boost your energy
C: Take your fatigue medications as ordered by your doctor
D: Use air conditioning and other cooling techniques

#129: **When teaching your MS patient who is experiencing fatigue, all of the following actions are appropriate except:**

A: Assessing the patient's mood, sleep habits, and encouraging regular rest periods, as needed.
B: Assessing the patient's environment for heat and humidity.
C: Encouraging the use of walkers, cane, wheelchair and other assistive devices, as needed.
D: Asking the patient to take warm baths, drink plenty of fluids, including caffein before bedtime.

#130: **Positive outcomes in the management of spasticity include all of the following except:**

A: Decreased clonus
B: Decreased spasms and stiffness
C: Decreased muscle hypertonia
D: Increased psychomotor function

#131: **All of the following statements are true about spasticity in MS except:**

A: Spasticity, exaggerated flexor reflexes and clonus occur in Multiple Sclerosis

B: Exacerbations, infections and noxious stimuli can heighten spasticity

C: Medications like Baclofen, Clonazepam, Tizanidine and Diazepam can be used to manage spasticity

D: Stretching of spastic muscles, use of warm or cold compresses are not helpful in managing muscle hypertonia.

#132: **A patient's quality of life would least likely be affected by which of the following?**

A: Speech and communication problems

B: Emotional and social isolation

C: Numbness and tingling sensations

D: Deteriorating cognitive ability

E: Difficulty ambulating

#133: **When addressing quality of life issues with MS patients, which of the following would be appropriate to do ?**

A: Be encouraging, supportive and empathetic.

B: Empower patients and facilitate adjustment to the diagnosis of MS.

C: Provide education, information and referral to appropriate resources.

D: Acknowledge that patients have varying desires and expectations.

E: All of the above

#134: **You are working with a 50 year old female who is on an injectable disease modifying agent for her Relapsing-remitting MS . She tells you the local furniture company she works for has filed for bankruptcy and she will lose her job in three months. The patient begins to cry, she is worried that if she loses this job she will not have health insurance to cover the cost of her medications. She tells you that losing her job will lead to financial hardship, and she may not be able to keep her current apartment if that happens. As the nurse you will:**

A: Refer the patient to a social worker at the Social Security Administration, for assistance with job training, job placement and possible Medicaid service.

B: Put the patient in touch with the case manager at the specific drug manufacturer, for possible patient assistance with her disease-modifying medication.

C: Give the patient information about the local unemployment office for financial assistance when her company closes.

D: Be supportive, assist the patient because you know interruptions in her medication management, plus financial and vocational constraints may affect her quality of life and her ability to live independently.

E: All of the above

#135: **Which of the following statement (s) describe (s) the (EDSS) Expanded Disability Status Scale?**

A: EDSS is a neurological assessment tool used to quantify disability and monitor changes in the level of disability in MS over a period of time.

B: It was developed in 1983 by a neurologist named John Kurtzke.

C: Walking and fatigability are the main disabilities measured in EDSS.

D: The EDSS is based on measurements of impairment in the eight components of the Functional Systems (FS)

E: All of the above

#136: **Your patient's score on the Expanded disability scale is 9.5. As the nurse you know that this patient's score indicate (s):**

A: He has no disability in his functional status and he is able to ambulate without any assistance.

B: He Is bedridden, totally dependent, has swallowing and speech difficulties.

C: He is at risk for aspiration, pressure ulcers and contractures.

D: B and C

#137: **Nursing research is important for all of the following except:**

A: Nurses gain new evidenced-based knowledge

B: Research helps guide nursing practice

C: Research provides support for the use of all new medications at the bedside

D: Research helps corroborate existing clinical knowledge

#138: Research is valid to nursing practice because of which of the following?

A: Nursing practice needs to be based on evidence.

B: Interpretation of research findings is utilized to facilitate patient and family education.

C: Use of evidenced-based research is important for validity and safety in nursing practice

D: a,b & c

#139: The Nurse's tasks and skills in research include:

A: Collection of samples in a proper manner

B: Having knowledge of research designs and its ethical principles

C: Working to increase nursing body of knowledge

D: Ensuring that proper preparation and documentation are in place

E: All of the above

140: **Which of the following definitions of clinical trial phases is not correct?**

A: Phase 1- Testing of side effects with increasing doses of a drug, to learn initial evidence of drug effectiveness. Determine the metabolism and pharmacological effects of a drug on about 20 to 100 enrolled volunteer subjects.

B: Phase 2- Testing of drug efficacy for a particular indication, watching for short term side effects and risks on about several hundred subjects with the same diagnoses.

C: Phase 3- Testing of drug therapeutics, efficacy, effectiveness and safety on about 1000 to 2000 people. Gathering of more evidence about the safety and effectiveness of the drug

D: Phase 4- Post marketing studies to monitor the drug's use by the public, to address issues brought by customers, to test product for uses by a different group or to make label changes to a product.

E: Phase 5-Doing follow up clinical trials on consumers who have had significant safety issues with the drug.

#141: Your Patient is scheduled to participate in a new clinical trial. About two hours before she was supposed to participate in the trial, she starts pacing around and informs you that she is worried because she does not really understand what the clinical trial is about. The best nursing action will be to:

A: Assure the patient that the doctors will make sure everything goes well.

B: Tell the patient not to worry, you are her nurse, you will watch over her through every step of the study process.

C: Find out if the patient has a signed consent form.

D: Notify the physician that the patient has not been given full informed consent

#142: Ethical nursing practice in MS includes all of the following except:

A: The nurse will maintain patient privacy and confidentiality, as per legal and regulatory guidelines and standards.

B: The nurse will be cognizant of issues related to age, culture, diversity and other issues, while providing care in a non-judgmental and non-discriminatory manner.

C: The nurse will deliver care in ways that maintain patient's rights, dignity, and autonomy.

D: The nurse will advocate for and make decisions for patients, so as to ensure that the right treatment modalities are implemented and adhered to.

#143: Which of the following are ethical principles that guide the MS nurse?

A: Beneficence and Nonmaleficence

B: Stewardship and justice

C: Autonomy and fidelity

D: All of the above

#144: **A middle age MS patient who is a subject in a clinical trial was given a narcotic for severe back pain not related to her MS. The patient's pain is controlled but she is now experiencing some confusion as a side effect of the narcotics. The patient's consent has not yet been signed. As a nurse you know that:**

A: Giving this patient the prescribed narcotics to manage her severe back pain is an act of beneficence.

B: Obtaining the consent when a patient is not in the appropriate cognitive state could result in possible maleficence.

C: Giving the patient the prescribed narcotics to manage her severe back pain, in a timely manner, is an act of stewardship and justice.

D: b and c

E: a and b

#145: **Which of the following statements about informed consent is not correct?**

A: The right of self determination and full disclosure are the ethical principles informed consents are based on.

B: Informed consents should include explanation of potential risks versus benefits of procedures, as well as disclosures about alternative options.

C: Informed consents must be explained in language that is easily understood by lay persons, and the subjects must be aware that they have the right to refuse all treatments and procedures without consequence.

D: The MS nurse is fully responsible for explaining all procedures and treatments informed consents are required for.

E: The MS nurse's role in facilitating informed consents, treatments and procedures includes, ensuring that MS patients and their families fully understand facts, benefits and risks before signing informed consent forms.

#146: **Which one of the following statements about MS is (are) true?**

A: Caucasians have a higher prevalence than Asians, Blacks or other ethnic groups living in the same geographical area.

B: MS prevalence rate is lower in Japan, but the disease prevalence is higher in Scandinavia and in people of Scandinavian descent.

C: Studies have shown that adolescents who migrate to lower prevalence areas before the age of 15 years acquire the lower risk of the new area they migrate to.

D: Adolescents who migrate after the age of 15 years maintain the MS risks of their place of birth.

E: E: All of the above

#147: **The MS nurse can strive towards getting professional development through all of the following except:**

A: Obtaining certification credentials, acting as a role model, preceptor and mentor.

B: Becoming a member of professional organizations such the IOMSN or other important organizations of MS nurses.

C: Having and maintaining knowledge and competency about MS nursing clinical practice, research and advocacy among other things.

D: Not adhering to the code of ethics and principles set by the American Nurses Association because that organization is not really very specific to MS nurses .

E: Becoming a writer, public speaker or support group leader.

#148: **Which one of the following will the MS nurse not consider doing when addressing psychosocial issues with MS patients and their families?**

A: Discuss Advanced Directives, encourage appropriate end of life planning.

B: Ensure that patients and their families have essential education, counseling and appropriate community agency referrals.

C: Avoid life planning discussions because those are personal patient and family issues.

D: Be a source of support and allow patients and families to verbalize their fears and concerns.

#149: **As a member of the comprehensive health team of Multiple Sclerosis care, the MS nurse knows that:**

A: MS is a chronic disease that is unpredictable, uncertain and has varying symptoms and prognosis from one individual to another.

B: The various symptoms and impairments that occur in MS are related to the demyelination and scarring of nerve fibers in the Central Nervous System.

C: These various impairments may be mild or severe, so patients have to learn to adapt to changes that may or may not impair their physical and functional abilities.

D: The nurse should encourage and promote patient empowerment, self-actualization and adherence to recommended care and treatment modalities.

E: All of the above

#150: **A newly diagnosed MS patient is having emotional problems and she tells you she feels stressed and overwhelmed about her diagnosis. All of the following are appropriate nursing interventions for this patient except:**

A: Tell the patient that there is no point in getting herself all stressed out, because she can't change the facts of her medical diagnosis.

B: Involve the social worker, encourage and promote referral for psychological counseling.

C: Discuss participation in support groups such as the National Multiple Sclerosis Society support group chapters.

D: Provide support and education for the patient, give information about credible MS online websites and other support networks.

Answers to Practice Questions

1. B
2. C
3. B
4. C
5. D
6. D
7. C
8. A
9. C
10. C
11. C
12. D
13. D
14. C
15. D
16. A
17. E
18. B
19. D
20. D
21. A
22. B
23. A
24. E
25. C
26. B
27. C
28. A
29. C
30. C
31. B
32. E
33. E
34. A
35. E
36. B

37. D
38. B
39. A
40. E
41. D
42. E
43. B
44. D
45. A
46. C
47. D
48. D
49. C
50. C
51. C
52. E
53. A
54. D
55. B
56. B
57. B
58. D
59. A
60. C
61. E
62. A
63. B
64. C
65. E
66. B
67. E
68. E
69. B
70. D
71. D
72. D
73. E
74. E

75. E
76. B
77. E
78. E
79. A
80. C
81. A
82. E
83. A
84. E
85. C
86. E
87. D
88. C
89. D
90. D
91. E
92. E
93. C
94. C
95. E
96. D
97. C
98. C
99. D
100.D
101.E
102.C
103.D
104.A
105.D
106.D
107.D
108.D
109.E
110.E
111.C
112.D

113.D
114.D
115.E
116.D
117.A
118.B
119.E
120.D
121.D
122.D
123.E
124.C
125.B
126.C
127.B
128.B
129.D
130.D
131.D
132.C
133.E
134.E
135.E
136.D
137.C
138.D
139.E
140.E
141.D
142.D
143.D
144.E
145.D
146.E
147.D
148.C
149.E
150.A

CONCLUSION

The Multiple Sclerosis Nursing International Certification Examination can be challenging.

I had to personally put together some solid test preparation and test taking techniques to help me PASS the Exam, at my very first attempt.

There is no doubt that certification examinations require good preparation and efforts from candidates. A combination of good study techniques and knowledge of critical test taking skills can be some of the best arsenals to help one pass these examinations.

Preparing and studying for certification exams require a lot of hard work and commitment on your part. As a nurse, your success in passing a certification exam, may bring you personal and professional benefits, but most importantly though, the patients you care for will have a certified nurse who has gained invaluable, critical knowledge that can translate into better Patient outcomes.

You are a nurse, your Patients' care and safety depend on your clinical knowledge, expertise, competence, dedication and compassion.

Do yourself and your patients a big favor, strive to be the best you can be. Get Certified!

Plan well. Do what needs to be done. Leave no stone unturned. Give it your all!

Believe in yourself! Be Confident! You are a Nurse! You got this! Go for it! Get Certified!

Nurses are life-long learners. Our patients depend and count on our expertise and knowledge as we provide care in our various clinical settings. We can all benefit from learning from one another. If you have any advice or suggestions that other colleagues can benefit from, please feel free to contact me at: adayans@gmail.com **or info@elitecarecorp.com**

Thank you for reading my book! **GOOD LUCK!**

Appendix A: Multiple Sclerosis Disease Modifying Medications

Injectable Medications

Rebif   (interferon beta-1a)

Avonex (interferon beta-1a)

Plegridy (Peginterferon beta-1a)

Rebif, **A**vonex, and **P**legridy are interferon beta-1a *(**M**nemonic:* **RAP**)

Betaseron

Extavia

Betaseron and Extavia are both
Interferon beta-1b **(Mnemonic: BE) 1b**

Glatopa (**Glatiramer acetat**e) is the generic version of Copaxone 20 mg dose.

Copaxone (**Glatirmer acetat**e) Copaxone comes in 20mg and 40mg doses.

ZINBRYTA (Daclizumab) :   FDA approved for Multiple Sclerosis treatment in May 2016.

Oral Medications

Tecfidera (Dimethyl fumarate)

Aubagio (Teriflunomide)

Gilenya   (Fingolimod)

Oral disease modifying agents —

Mnemonic:- (**_TAG_**)

Intravenous Medications

Lemtrada   (Alemtuzumab)

Novantrone (Mitoxantrone)

Tysabri   (Natalizumab)

 LiNT,silent i,for IV meds reminder,
or
MAN   for **M**itoxantrone, **A**lemtuzumab, **N**atalizumab.

Appendix: B: Online Resources

Multiple Sclerosis Nurses International Certification Board: http://www.msnicb.org

International Organization of Multiple Sclerosis Nurses: http://www.iomsn.org

Consortium of Multiple Sclerosis Centers: http://www.mscare.org

MS Views and News: http://www.msviews.org

National Multiple Sclerosis Society(NMSS) http://www.nmss.org

Multiple Sclerosis Association of America (MSAA) http://www.msaa.com

Multiple Sclerosis International Federation: http://www.msif.org

Multiple Sclerosis Foundation (MSF) http://www.msfocus.org

Multiple Sclerosis Awareness Foundation (MSAF) : http://www.msawareness.org

Can Do Multiple Sclerosis: http://www.mscando.org

The Myelin Project USA: http://www.myelin.org

MS World: http://www.msworld.org

www.actharmsrelapse.com

www.RethinkMSRelapses.com

Appendix: C: Pharmaceutical Companies

Teva (Glatiramer Acetate/ Copaxone): www.copaxone.com

Serono (Rebif): http://mslifelines.com

Accorda (Dalfampradine; Ampyra): http://www.ampyra.com

Novatis (Extavia; Interferon beta-1b; Fingolimod/ Gilenya): http://www.extavia.com

Sanofi Genzyme (alentuzumab/ Lemtrada): http://www.lemtrada.com

Biogen (Natalizumab/Tysabri, Dymethylfumarate /Tecfidera, Zinbryta) http://www.tysabri.com

References

Halper, June., & Harris Colleen. (2012). Nursing Practice in Multiple Sclerosis: A Core Curriculum (3rd ed). New York, NY: Springer
Publishing Company

Halper, June,. & Holland, N.J. (2011). Comprehensive Nursing Care In Multiple Sclerosis (3rd ed). New York, NY: Springer Publishing Company

Birnbaum, G. L. (2013). Multiple Sclerosis: Clinician's Guide to Diagnosis and Treatment
New York, NY: Oxford University Press

Macaluso, V. F. (2015). Multiple Sclerosis From Both Sides of the Desk.
Bloomington, IN: IUniverse

Brorsen, A.J,. & Rogelet, K.R (2014). Adult CCRN Certification Review
Burlington, MA: Jones & Bartlett Learning

Sheremata, W.A. (2011).100 Questions & Answers About Multiple Sclerosis (2nd ed.)
Sudbury, MA: Jones & Bartlett Learning

Made in the USA
Monee, IL
08 May 2023

33318592R00046